Pre-School

Training

Everything Modern Parents Need to

Know about Potty Training to Do It

Right

Regina Williams

ISBN: 978-1-63750-223-5

Table of Contents

PRE-SCHOOLER POTTY TRAINING 1

INTRODUCTION 6

CHAPTER 1...8

WHAT'S POTTY TRAINING ALL ABOUT? 8

CHAPTER 2...13

POTTY TRAINING READINESS 13

Getting Ready to Kick-Start potty Training 14

Duration for Learning Potty Training 18

Parenting Factor for Potty Decisions 19

Basic Essentials for Potty Training a Child...20

CHAPTER 3...22

POTTY TRAINING BENEFICIAL FACT 22

CHAPTER 4...28

MEASURES TO TAKE BEFORE STARTING POTTY TRAINING 28

Ensuring Toddler's Readiness 29

Make Your Child Identify the Act...30

Ensure Your Strategies are Natural 31

Teach Your Toddler the Language...32

Effect of Demonstrations during Training 34

Carefully Select Your Potty Words! 36

Promote Your Son or Daughter's Independence 38

CHAPTER 5...40

POTTY TRAINING 40

How to Determine Your Potty-Training Strategy 41

How to Enhance Potty Training Success...44

CHAPTER 6 ....**48**

MATERIALS FOR POTTY TRAINING A CHILD 48

A Portable Potty Seat 48

Potty Location 51

Training Pants 53

CHAPTER 7 ....**55**

POTTY TRAINING STRATEGIES 55

Take Things Slowly 56

No Clothing Approach 56

Dressing for Training Course 59

Bed-time Approach 61

Training Pants or Disposables (Diapers)? 62

Having Realistic Expectations 63

Making Potty Training Child-Friendly 64

CHAPTER 8 ....**66**

READING BODY SIGNS FOR POTTY ACT 66

CHAPTER 9 ....**71**

ETHICS OF POTTY TRAINING 71

Get Him or Her to Jump to Start with Indicators 71

Be Prepared to Reach a Toilet Quickly 72

Potty Prize Giving Approach 74

Relax when Accidents Occur 76

Offer Reward to Enhance Potty Learning 78

Duration of Encouragement 79

Patience 80

CHAPTER 10 ....**82**

BED WETTING 82

How to Know When to Stop Using Diaper 86

How to Enhance Toddler Dryness *87*

CHAPTER 11 ....**92**

MOST COMMONLY KNOWN REASONS FOR POTTY TRAINING PROBLEMS 92

CHAPTER 12 ....**96**

BEHAVIOURAL INFLUENCE ON POTTY TRAINING 96

DEDICATION **112**

Introduction

This training on potty learning is the perfect training program for your child. With the strategies explained, it is easy for your little one to handle potty independently. This training on potty is suitable for babies, toddler, and kids.

In this pioneering, practical book, parenting expert *Regina Williams* offers a revolutionary approach to child parenting with key strategies that foster healthy brain development, leading to calmer, happier children successful with potty learning. She explains—and make accessible—the new science of how a child's brain is wired and how it matures enough to handle potty activity efficiently and independently. The brain in young children, the right brain and its emotions tend to rule over the logic of the left brain, which is why effective potty-training strategy is required for effective potty learning. By applying these ultimate strategies and discoveries to everyday parenting, you can turn any outburst, argument, or fear into a chance to integrate your child's brain and foster vital growth.

This Potty training book is designed to help your children learn how to use the toilet bowl with confidence, keeping them secure and comfortable. The Author *Regina Williams* is a perfect potty trainer for little boys and girls.

Chapter 1

What's Potty training All About?

At the beginning of the grand experience of teaching a child to use the potty, many parents question how they'll ever accomplish such a complicated task. They watch their toddler with his brand-new potty dish on his head playing and questioning the sanity that persuaded them as a parent to buy the potty initially. The glad tidings are that almost all children can get better at daytime toilet/potty training at age three (3) to five (5) roughly, and for some families, it's a pleasant, even fun experience.

Take the time to think about how exactly you teach your son or daughter another new lease of life skills. How will you teach your son or daughter to recite the alphabet, draw a picture, tie up his or her shoelace, dress him or herself, or come up with a puzzle?

Do you spend one full day on extreme non-formal lessons or teaching for your kids and then expect your son or daughter to pass the test by the end of the day? Would you demand that he or she show mastery every day after that without ever making any errors?

I question it! If you do approach lessons in this manner, you'd likely finish up frustrated as well as your child would maintain tears.

The actual way that people teach children new skills is by carrying it out gradually, over days, weeks, celebrating every little victory that follows. This won't apply merely to toddlers, it's a design you'll follow as an adult for quite some time too, which include your son or daughter; from the first new experience on riding bicycle, to the very first time on skis, to the new level of driving a car, and in regards to a million other new things we all do.

Considering your part in your son or daughter's learning processes, how will you strategize when teaching your son or daughter something new?

Are you going to be extreme and psychological?

Would you demand that he sit down still and give consideration?

Would you put a crayon in his hands and demand that he start painting when you sit down and get worried that he'll never figure out how to draw a compelling picture or print a capital A?

Would you consider yourself seated next to him, taking records when he would get to a better level?

Would you fret that he'll be putting on Velcro sneakers to senior high school or you need to button his tux for him on his big day?

Obviously not! You understand that your son or daughter will get good at these skills and many more during his or her lifetime, which teaching him or her is one of your jobs as a mother or father.

Think about your expectations when teaching your son or daughter something new. When teaching him to draw an image of the family, what do you anticipate to be the very first thing he'll deposit on paper? A family group portrait? No, it's a scribble! And you will take pleasure in his work and post his artwork on the refrigerator door. As time passes, and with repetition, that scribble will need shape till your son or daughter will pull circles and squares and soon homes, people, and pets.

Now let look at this next new event in your son or daughter's life: *Potty/Toilet training.* You should be able to strategize potty training in the same manner that you do every other new skill step-by-step, as time passes, with pleasure, kindness, and endurance. Let discuss those essential strategies needed to ensure smooth potty training.

Chapter 2

Potty Training Readiness

You can start potty training a kid at any age: you can even set a new baby on the potty bowl. However, *the most crucial question is; when will the training be finished?* A kid will complete potty/toilet training when his biology, skills, and development have matured to a spot that he's able and willing to dominate complete control of his toileting. Only then can he or she recognizes the necessity to stop his or her game, go directly to the toilet, handle the whole process, and go back to his or her game.

The quantity of time it requires for your son or daughter to understand toilet training is closely related to the span between your commencement of the training and the strategies applied; few months old when you begin training and when he or she is physically and emotionally in a position to take responsibility. Several studies also show that no matter when the potty or toilet training starts, nearly all children are just physically endowed with the capacity of 3rd party toileting after age group two, and mastery usually happens between age range two (2) and four (4).

Getting Ready to Kick-Start potty Training

Not only will it be that you don't need to hurry the procedure, simply because rushing things can result in a disaster. It places incredible stress on both you and your child. It makes the complete process a miserable experience rather than the normal learning process that it ought to be. A lot more, when stress and pressure enter the picture, it can create tantrums, constipation, extreme mishaps, and setbacks.

Your son or daughter will figure out how to use the toilet. She'll learn best in her way and on her time plan. There is absolutely no award for the most quickly trained child. And research proves again that early or past due toileting mastery has nothing at all whatsoever regarding how smart or intelligent a kid is.

A kid can be placed on the toilet bowl even while still a child, and in a few cultures, this is routinely done. A little percentage of American and Canadian parents have followed this practice, called EC. Before you subscribe to thinking your daily life just got a lot easier, you should know that EC is not toilet training. It is a long-lasting, soft, gradual system that can be used rather than diapers to control a child's waste materials. It replaces hourly diaper changes with hourly trips to the toilet.

With this technique, parents read their baby's body language and sound cues to put her on the toilet container when they believe that it is time on her behalf to defecate. The mother or father manages the child's defecation process before the child is mature with the capacity of total individual toileting, which often happens at the age range mentioned previously: from two to four years old.

If the thought of changing diapers with the strategy of watching your son or daughter's body signals and putting him or her on the potty suits you, then research one of the numerous books on this issue known as EC. In this toilet training book, we'll strategize toilet training from the more prevalent toddler-readiness approach.

For the vast majority of families who consider toilet training a toddler event, some can look for a fast-fix solution. However, even those interesting books or programs that guarantee one-day results have a significant stipulation: they recommend using the ideas only once a kid shows all the symptoms of readiness and reaches a starting age group of about 2yrs. Besides, they warn that unfortunate incidents might occur for weeks afterward, and the mother or father must be diligent in taking the kid to the toilet regularly.

Duration for Learning Potty Training

When toilet/potty training starts at about age group two, it can take from three (3) months to a year of toilet training before the child gains potty independence. Generally, the younger the kid is, the fewer readiness skill she possesses; the greater a mother or father must be engaged, and the much longer chance of success would take.

Regardless of your method of toilet training, 98% of children are completely independent by age four. (Nighttime dryness is another issue, predicated on physiology, and may take a lot longer.)

Parenting Factor for Potty Decisions

Toilet/potty training isn't just an all or nothing decision. Many parents start the procedure early with the youngster because they might instead assist, remind, and tidy up a few mishaps than continue steadily to change diapers. Some decide to begin by slowly watching their child's body signals to advance to each new level. Others concentrate intently on strategies with expectations to make things work swiftly.

Any path you select for your baby can work, as long as you are positive and patient. Regardless of your plan, it can help to go from diapers to total self-reliance. For most parents, halfway is not a bad spot to be, even if indeed they spend half a year at that midpoint.

Parenting is filled up with choices, and the ultimate decisions are incredibly different for each family. There is not just one single right to toilet train or potty train a child; the methods are extensive. The right strategy for you is the one that feels convenient to you and works for you as well as your child. Eventually, you will have to assess what your loved one's goals are and then arranged an idea that is most effective for you.

Basic Essentials for Potty Training a Child

There can be an enormous market for potty training paraphernalia, such as expensive dolls that soak and wet, specially made toilet chair, tot-sized urinals, fancy charts, posters, prizes, and awards. While many of these can easily make for a great experience, it isn't in any way necessary to buy a range of products for such a very simple, natural process.

A potty chair, twelve pairs of training jeans, and a relaxed and enjoyable ambiance of learning are what's needful to teach your son or daughter how to use the toilet or potty. Anything extra is optional.

Chapter 3

Potty Training Beneficial Fact

You probably don't believe much about your potty process, and it's probably so because the color and uniformity of your son or daughter's diaper deposits have been part of your daily activities. There are a few facts that are beneficial to know as you attempt the potty/toilet training journey.

- Potty training has nothing in connection with nighttime dryness. Nighttime dryness is achieved only once a child's physiology facilitates it. A kid bed-wets while asleep due to some amount of reasons: his kidneys aren't sending a sign to his brain when he's asleep to alert him he must go pee or poo, his bladder hasn't yet grown large enough to accommodate urine all night, his bladder overproduces urine at night time, or he sleeps so deeply that he doesn't stay awake to visit the toilet. As children develop, many of these conditions are personally corrected. This usually occurs between the age range of three (3) and six (6). This is not something you can educate, and you can't rush it.

- *A parent's readiness to teach is as crucial as a child's readiness to learn.* A kid can't understand how to use the toilet unless someone shows him or her. As well as the teacher's strategy and attitude can have a direct impact on how long the procedure takes and exactly how pleasurable the journey would be. A parent who is stressed about the process or who's too busy to dedicate enough time necessary for teaching can gradually complicate the procedure, or even take it to a screeching halt. Conversely, an educated, patient mother or father with a pleasurable strategy can make the process pleasurable and bring far better, and quicker result.

- Most toddlers urinate four to eight times every day, usually about every two hours roughly. A child's bladder can hold one and a half ounces of urine for every year old. (A two-year-old's bladder can take about 2-3 ounces; a three-year-old's, around 3 to 4.5 ounces; and a four-year-old's, about 4-6 ounces-less when compared to a cup.)

- Most toddlers have a couple of bowel patterns every day; some have three, while others neglect a day or two among patterns. Generally, each young one has a regular pattern.

- A child's diet will influence the total amount and frequency of urination and bowel motions. Adequate daily liquids, including drinking water, plus a nutritious diet comprising foods with a lot of fiber (fruits, vegetables, and wholegrain) can make reduction easier, which subsequently makes toilet training more comfortable.

- Ample daily exercise means that your son or daughter's stool is shifted through her system correctly. Insufficient movement can lead to constipation.

- A child's pelvic and sphincter muscles need to relax to be able to release a pee or poop. Stress, pressure, or panic is a surefire way to avoid the procedure. (That is why some children use their diaper soon after they are coming out of the toilet.).

- Polls show that more than 80 percent of parent say that their children experience some set back in toilet training. This high number indicates that what we often label as "setbacks" is just the most common way to mastery of toileting. Exactly like any new thing that children learn, it isn't always a smooth process from beginning to end. It's similar to a squiggly range, with bursts of success as well as nags and pauses on the way to the ultimate result.

- It doesn't seem to really matter what strategy can be used for toilet teaching/potty training, because

98% of children are entirely time-independent at age group four (4).

CHAPTER 4

Measures to Take before Starting Potty Training

When kids learn a new skill, they rarely learn it all at one time. Typically, they process the information in manageable pieces. You have to believe and understand how your son or daughter learn to process and respond to information. The process began in the past when he was a child and learned to carry up his mind and shoulders and also to control his body. He progressed to sitting down, after that to crawling, and to walking while you hold him by hand. Shortly he was cruising the home furniture. After a period, he took those initial shaky steps, as soon as those were perfected, he began to walk. This organic sequence of occasions took from ten to twenty weeks.

Just as that you patiently and methodically helped your son or daughter learn to do things naturally, you can motivate him to understand the countless details involved in potty training before you actively start potty training, that can do a lot of things that set your son or daughter up for catching up with the learning process when it's high time.

Ensuring Toddler's Readiness

Most kids enjoy books and like to be read to. Many great children's books, created precisely for toddlers, can be found on potty training. Make an effort to get those books which have photographs of kids with books that make use of colorful pictures of pets and likely creatures learning how exactly to use the toilet.

Reading these books before training can help your son or daughter become familiar with the theory in a fun, non-threatening way without expectations attached. You can even make use of these same books as potty-time reading when teaching begins.

Make Your Child Identify the Act

Each time you change your son or daughter's diaper, you have an opportunity to train a bit about elimination. Making casual comments about elimination is an excellent method to teach. Take for instance, *"You have poopoo in your diaper."* Or, *"Your diaper is wet because you peed. Mommy pees in the potty."*

A few brief explanations as time passes are helpful. You can clarify that the wetness is pee-pee and the dark brown stuff is poopoo. Inform him or her that they are leftovers that her body doesn't need. Explain a clean, dried out diaper is a lot nicer to wear.

Help your child recognize what's taking place when you see that she's wetting or filling her diaper:

Luckily for you, if you capture her tinkling in the toilet bowl or if you feel that unexpected warmth in her diaper while carrying her. At this period you can explain what she's carrying out and let her understand that in a period like that she'll learn to perform it in the potty.

Ensure Your Strategies are Natural

Babies and also toddlers accept things that happen in their diaper as normal and natural. It is not until siblings, peers, and adults instruct them there's some factor disgusting about these procedures that they think in another case. Try to let your son or daughter maintain this innocent view-point about elimination. This can help toilet teaching, and potty training becomes a more definite knowledge without any embarrassment or shame.

Don't attach negative worth to wet or messy diapers. (Ensure you avoid words like miserable, icky, stinky or smelly) Do not make a significant creation about the smell or consistency, and do your very best to caution your son or daughter's big brothers and sisters about this!

Teach Your Toddler the Language

Throughout your everyday events, coach your toddler, the phrases and meanings of toilet-related terminologies such as body parts, urination, bowel motions, and toilet duties. When enough time comes for real potty schooling, there is so very much to learn, so that it will be useful if he or she currently is more comfortable with the necessary information.

Lots of terms that are used during potty training aren't directly toilet-related but can make different concepts for your son or daughter to comprehend. Descriptive words that you'll use during the procedure are those like wet, dry, clean, flush, and toilet paper (tissue paper).

Teach your child the idea of opposites and specific purposes which will give a foundation for toilet training. Wet/dried out, on/off, messy/clean, up/down, stop/proceed, now/later, these are concepts that'll be part of the potty training routine.

It's common for parents to employ a mixture of phrases and terms during the potty process, but doing this can confuse a fresh trainee. If for instance, you question him if he would "go potty," however, the next day you asked him "to go use the toilet," and later consult him if he must "tinkle," he might not follow your school of thought. It is best if you choose your vocabulary conditions and adhere to them during the training process.

Effect of Demonstrations during Training

It can be beneficial to let your child see you or her siblings utilize the toilet. You won't need to have her view every detail; it's much enough to have her discover you take a seat on the toilet bowl while you explain what you are doing. Tell her that whenever she gets heavily pressed, she'll place her pee-pee and poo-poo in the toilet, too, rather than in her diaper.

If your son or daughter has older siblings, cousins, or friends, tell her that they used diapers when they were her age, however now they utilize the toilet. If they're available to accompany in the toilet, let your baby get a glimpse of his or her sibling or peer using the potty. Allow her to understand that when she gets just a little older, she'll produce that act too.

Don't assume all parent is ready to have little eye viewing while they utilize the toilet, and it's not essential for you to do that if you like your privacy, teach your son or daughter to respect a shut bathroom and toilet door. Remember that as your son or daughter masters her very own toileting, she is more likely to stick to your footsteps and desire her privacy as well. Set up the toilet so that it's safe and sound and manageable on her behalf, and keep hearing open when she is alone in the toilet.

Carefully Select Your Potty Words!

Certain words are normal in particular geographic areas, plus some are more trusted than others. If you pay attention to daycare, the recreation center, or the retail shopping center, you'll soon know very well what words are normally used in town.

Here are a few of the words most used by families with small children:

Body Terms: Urination, bowel movement, vulva (everything you can see) and vagina (the canal inside), penis, buttocks/rectum, flatulence.

Family Words: Toilet, pot, potty, privy, loo pee, pee-pee, move potty, go pee-pee, tinkle, pissy, wee-wee, go wee, wee, wees, tee-tee, visit the bathroom, visit the toilet, utilize the potty, go (as in, "will you go?") poop, poopie, poo-poo, poos, caca, BM, move poo-poo, number two, utilize the potty, vulva, vagina, privates, bottom level, girl parts, penis, willy bottom level, bum, tush, toches/tucks, cheeks, fanny, behind, buns, rear gas, passing gas, passing wind, fart*, toot, breaking wind, blow off, poot, fluffer, stinker, etc. are regarded a rude term for children in a few families but regular in others.

Certain scientific or specialized terminologies sound odd when used with a kid. Can you envisage yourself asking your baby, *"Have you got pressure in your rectum indicating that you need to defecate?"* Instead, choose words that you'd be comfortable having your son or daughter use and understand fast. Use whatever phrases with which your loved ones is preferred and familiar; remember that these words will likely be called or used by your child in a general public place, so it is safer to adhere to socially acceptable language.

Promote Your Son or Daughter's Independence

This is the time to encourage your son or daughter to do things on her behalf, for example; putting on her socks, draw up her pants, remove her jacket, carry a plate to the desk, and climb directly into her car seat. All of these tasks nurture a sense of independence, which will be essential for potty mastery.

As your son or daughter masters each task, her degree of confidence will develop. The more she can perform, the more she'll be ready to try. Each achievement builds on previous successes, as well as your child will discover herself to be someone who can try brand new things and be proficient at performing them. This attitude will become especially helpful when it's to introduce potty training.

CHAPTER 5

Potty Training

Having decided that the time is here to commence potty and toilet training, your son or daughter is ready and you're prepared. So, what's next?

Firstly, ensure that your attitude and expectations are in the best place. You ought to be feeling calm and positive. It's also advisable to understand that the training process may take as long as half a year or more, so forget about any hope you may have to toilet train your toddler in merely a day. Exactly like learning how to walk, chat, or take beverage from a cup, understanding how to utilize the toilet bowl, and really should end up being a gradual, pleasurable experience for you both.

Before you place a potty in the toilet, it is time to create your supplies and execute a little planning. Below are the necessary measures to take.

How to Determine Your Potty-Training Strategy

There isn't just one single best way to potty train a child. There are various approaches that can lead you to success. As you make decisions about how exactly to begin this grand endeavor, have a few things to consider:

- What is your son or daughter's learning design? How has he or she learned various other new skills? Will he or she observe and absorb before she tackles something? Or will he or she dive in and function her method through it? Is he or she a thoughtful listener or a hands-on doer?

- What exactly do you do that mostly motivates him or her to try something new? What activities bring the best outcomes? Is your enthusiasm more than enough to get your child to try something new? Or what activities do you perform to convince and persuade him or her before he or she will test it out? Will he or she do anything his or her old sibling or cousin will?

- What's your teaching design and strategy? Do you describe verbally before you display? Do you present it step-by-step with commentary? Do you perform by gently demonstrating? Do you set items up and allow your child to find out what's happening by himself?

- How much time have you got to potty train your child? Are you available all day together with your kid or home only at a specific time of the day? Will you devote an uninterrupted chunk of the period to get started, accompanied by snippets of time each day afterward? Or are you considering fitting training into your already busy schedule?

- What are your targets? What do you consider would be much easier for you: changing diapers or assisting your son or daughter on the potty? Would you instead concentrate intently on potty schooling for two weeks and move issues along? Or do you read articles to teach and train while you let your son or daughter set the speed, mastering one stage at a time?

- Who'll be the teachers? Do you want to potty train by yourself? Or will several people be involved in the training?

Most of these issues can affect the toilet/potty training experience. Taking time to examine these points can help you plan the best strategy for you, your son or daughter, and the others of your loved ones, too.

How to Enhance Potty Training Success

Whether you are employing elimination communication with a three-month-old, pre-training an eighteen-month-old, or introducing a brand-new concept to a three-year-old, there are two important factors that may affect the process above all, both of these factors will establish the pace for potty training. These could make the toilet schooling journey a demanding, unpleasant event, or even ensure that it is an excellent, successful process.

These two factors could make your son or daughter miserable or make him or her content. They can make any strategy an unexpected disaster, or they can make nearly every potty/toilet training method work beautifully.

What exactly are these excellent factors? *The teacher's attitude and the teacher's degree of patience.*

Allow me to say this again to ensure that you grasp this essential concept. *Both factors which will set the speed* *for potty training effectiveness are your **attitude as well as your patience**.*

You'll remember that I didn't mention anything about the mentee or student! That's because kids learn factors from their parents and other folks in their life, which is what they practice. And kids are like small sponges. Children are continually watching others, specifically the adults in their life. They grab cues from others about how exactly they should respond in a variety of situations; whether it's the first time on an equine, the first flavor of papaya or the first take a seat on a potty chair, your child will end up being learning from you.

So, no matter where your son or daughter is in the readiness department, and regardless of what approach you choose to take, be sure that these factors are in proper place before starting potty training process.

The two important indicators for effective and successful toilet schooling process popularly known as potty training are;

i.   The teacher's positive and supportive attitude.

ii. The teacher's kind and understanding tolerance.

CHAPTER 6

Materials for Potty Training a Child

You need to have all you need at hand before starting the potty teaching process. The information below would help you make your grocery list for potty training process.

A Portable Potty Seat

No matter what sort of toilet arrangement you possess at home, it's likely that your son or daughter will end up being facing a different circumstance when he or she's away. It's beneficial to purchase a chair adjuster that you could retain in your purse or diaper handbag. Which is a folding you can use when you're abroad. It adapts larger toilets to your son or daughter's size and makes them a bit more familiar, which is usually essential for brand-new trainees who are convenience-able with just a little potty in the home but could be overwhelmed or frightened by a large toilet and stall in an open public place.

It's wise to apply this lightweight adjuster in the home a few moments before going out. Otherwise, it's as unfamiliar as the unusual toilet you are putting it upon.

A normal adult toilet doesn't fit a kid very well. It's hard to climb up to it, and a child must balance and hold himself up while seated, making elimination more challenging. The hole usually is large enough for a tyke to fall through into the water, which may be a frightening encounter for a child. An improved choice for a fresh trainee can be a child-sized potty or an adapter potty chair insert along with a sturdy footstool.

There are many types available, so check around online store. A child-sized seat or chair is certainly essential to help significantly provide the toilet right down to your son or daughter's size and make it friendly, secure, and manageable. Almost any type will work, and the decision is yours.

Some potty seats have a high, removable splash safeguard created to prevent a fresh trainee from splattering the toilet. While the purpose for these is ordinarily useful plus they can serve the reason, splash guards also present a personal injury hazard. Many kids lose their balance in the process.

Potty Location

If you are utilizing a potty chair rather than an insert, you

can stick it wherever you would like. Many households

place the potty in the toilet right beside the big toilet. The

benefit to this is that your son or daughter gets

accustomed to the location, and it creates access for easy

dumping and washing. It also helps a kid connect the

potty with the actions that follow because other members

of the family use the toilet in the same space.

The disadvantage to maintaining your child's potty close

to the toilet is that if your toilet is quite a few distances

away from the places in your house where your son or

daughter spends his or her time, you might have several

accidents initially while he or she is on the path to the

toilet. This will stop, however, as your son or daughter gets utilized to reading his body signs.

Some families decide to keep the potty seat in the area where the kid spends time mostly. Throughout the day, it could be kept in your lobby. If you do that, it's wise to create a small potty nook or part to permit a child, therefore, have privacy and to reinforce the idea that this is not a public event. Through the bedtime routine and overnight, the potty could be kept in the bedroom for easy access, if you'd like. The benefit of a portable potty is definitely that your son or daughter is most likely to access the potty in time. The drawback is definitely that at some time, you will have to transfer your son or daughter's urine or feces to the toilet, but most children get this to change easily after they are potty trained.

Training Pants

Get a way to obtain a dozen or even more cotton training pants or a few boxes of disposable pull-up trousers. These will herald the brand new stage of advancement for your child and become a clear transmission that something fresh has begun.

Thick absorbent training jeans (instead of regular underwear) are excellent for new trainees. They'll absorb most or all your child's accidents and protect your floors and furniture.

Disposable pull-up pants are a well-known choice for brand-new trainees. Take note, however, that the disposables can backfire (as they say). Because they may feel like diapers to your child, your child may deal with them as such. Consider among the new types that certainly are a little much less unwieldy and also have an obtain-wet liner which allows your son or daughter to feel the wetness, which can only help him to recognize, and ideally avoid wet sense.

Children can change to less bulky and more attractive underwear after they start to show some improvement.

CHAPTER 7

Potty Training Strategies

Once you've decided about how you'll approach potty training with your kid and gathered all of your supplies, it's nearly time to start the process actively. Following are a few points to consider as you progress.

Keep in mind the two miracle factors; *the teacher's excellent attitude and kind patience will set the pace for the toilet or potty-training journey.* Take a breath, relax, and appreciate the knowledge with your baby.

Take Things Slowly

If you feel relaxed about the procedure, it's likely your son or daughter will as well. Ironically, the much less you push, the quicker the outcomes will occur.

The more you hurry, the much longer it will require. Even if a day time or an additional deadline looms, don't hurry the process with an excessive amount of strength and pressure. Being even more relaxed can help your child find out more conveniently and will get this to be less demanding for you too.

No Clothing Approach

If you're fortunate to begin training in warm weather, or when you can turn heat up in your house during training, hold your toddler in only training pants for a week roughly. Children often resist coping with ON/OFF requirement during teaching, since it takes so very much time and effort based on their limited skills. Therefore, the less clothing to cope with, the better!

Some parents let their children roam naked during training, but it isn't for everyone. Consider it before you bring in the theory to your baby, because he or she is more likely to like the freedom and could surprise you by carrying out a bit more of it than you expect. You might want to consider your family's method of nudity. How are things managed during bath time? How can you respond if your son or daughter walks in when you are dressing? If your family culture is certainly one of modesty and you suddenly let your son or daughter roam the home naked, it could send him or her some complicated mixed messages.

However, some families are even more relaxed about your body's natural state. Kids, siblings, and parents bathe jointly, toddlers play in the toilet as Mommy showers and dresses, and little males potty trained while peeing alongside Daddy. If this describes your family style, then you might look for a small extra time to help your child tune in with her body's elimination process.

One of the various other things to take into account here is that whenever using the naked strategy, all those early mishaps (among several others) will be unhindered by clothes and property unprotected wherever your son or daughter might be, and it will not be his or her fault or whatever you can prevent. For those who have carpeting or home furniture that may be ruined by accidents, you may take working out of the backyard or choose to go the almost naked approach instead and pop a set of training jeans on your little one.

Dressing for Training Course

It's more challenging for a toddler to get to the toilet in time but having the complication of snaps, zippers, and buttons. Many a trainee managed to get to the toilet and then have a major accident standing before the toilet, wanting to undress. For another couple of months and probably actually longer, your son or daughter should, whenever possible, avoid wearing pants with buttons, snaps, belts, or zippers and T-shirts that hang beneath the waist. Be sure that your son or daughter can remove her clothes easily and quickly. Regarding dresses, get them short more than enough to be able to remove them completely and well taken care of.

The very best clothing for a fresh potty trainee is a T-shirt and shorts or slacks with an elastic waistband. Make certain these are relatively loose fit so that your son or daughter can easily have them up and down.

At the start of training, you might want to have your son or daughter actually remove his or her trousers and underwear when he or she uses the potty, because there are a great number of new things to consider and having a wad of jeans around his or her ankles could be distracting and partially lowered slacks can become splattered. If you do not have him remove his trousers, feel absolute to help him consider his clothing off and place them back on, also if he can perform it himself. Needing to dress and undress in about ten situations a day will work fast for a dynamic toddler and may result in disinterest in using the potty at all. Don't worry, though he or she will adapt to this section of the process very quickly.

Bed-time Approach

Many children will remain in nighttime diapers for a year or much longer after daytime achievement. Nighttime dryness is attained only once a child's biology facilitates this, you can't hurry it, so don't also try. (Occasional bed-wetting is known as normal until approaching age six.)

Maintain a routine of placing diapers or disposable pull-up on your kid for naps or bedtime. The moment he or she is awake, remove it and also have him or her utilize the potty because so many children will eliminate soon after getting up. Switch your son or daughter out of nighttime diapers when the morning hours diaper is regularly dry.

Training Pants or Disposables (Diapers)?

Once your child gets a general idea and has started having daily success on the potty, you might want to change from diapers or disposable pull-up to cloth teaching pants to make things go along even faster.

The drawback to thickly padded disposable diapers or super-absorbent training pants is that they disguise wetness so very much that your son or daughter probably isn't bothered about it, whereas cotton training pants, or disposables with a stay-wet liner, signal wetness immediately and aren't extremely comfortable to wear when wet or messy. This can help your child to be more alert to what's happening down there.

Also, be sure you keep your son or daughter's pants a little loose so your baby can pull them easily. Training slacks or pull-ups ought to be a size larger than necessary. You desire them to be manageable for your son or daughter, without being so big that they droop.

Having Realistic Expectations

Understanding how to master toileting is normally a huge task for just a little child (kids). Mastery comes into play with time and patience. Sometimes will be more effective in some children than others. Sometimes when the house is tranquil and the day to day routine is definitely in place, your son or daughter will significantly have more success.

Making Potty Training Child-Friendly

Can your child easily open the door and turn on the light? Reach the toilet paper? Get right up to the sink? If he or she is facing difficulty addressing and using her potty, she'll be less thinking about using it routinely. Also, if she counts on you to perform everything on her behalf, you'll be passing up on a wonderful facet of potty teaching: encouraging your son or daughter's independence is vital.

Many small children are suspicious of empty rooms, and several fear the dark. There is nothing scarier compared to the cavern of a dark toilet. Through the training months, and perhaps actually for an extended period after schooling, accept that you'll either need to accompany your kid each time or keep the way and toilet carefully well to chase apart any unwanted shadows.

Chapter 8

Reading Body Signs for Potty Act

Understanding your child's body signal for potty activities enable you to help him or her get to the toilet fast.

The following are some typically common signals of an imminent bowel movement:

- Timing (very first thing each morning or ten to thirty minutes after a meal).

- Passing-by repeatedly.

- Squatting.

- Touching diaper.

- Tensed facial expression.

- Grunting.

- Stopping active play.

- Bending forward while holding tummy.

- Stomach-ache.

And below are a few common signals of impending urination:

- Timing (very first thing on awakening each morning or after a nap, one and half hour (1.5hrs) to two hours (2hrs) after last pee, or twenty (20) to forty-five minutes (45mins) after drinking).

- Holding crotch.

- Sitting on heels.

- Crossing legs.

- Squeezing thighs together.

- Squirming and wiggling (the potty dance).

- Bouncing.

- Shifting from feet to foot.

- Rocking backward and forwards.

- Becoming still and motionless.

- Whimpering.

The most crucial thing to bear in mind is that it is their (kids) accomplishment and milestone, not yours as a parent. **It is important to be sensitive to their timeline.**

The more we support them in having their success and their very own accomplishment (with only a small amount of psychological attachment on our side), the quicker the achievement and the more pleasant the knowledge for kids and parents!

When your child's day to day routine is disrupted or when he's overtired, hungry, or overstimulated, he'll likely have significantly more accidents and become more forgetful in what he or she is said to be doing.

Teaching your kid how to utilize the toilet is unarguably a permanent lesson. Between dried outruns and real potty calls, you will probably find yourself accompanying him to the toilet up to a dozen times a day! That results in 84 times support to the toilet over a week and some 360 times per month!

One method to keep perspective is to write down the starting day of potty teaching and note another time of about 90 days to the future. Understand that you'll end up being your kid's potty partner for at least those 90 days.

Remember, it could take typically three (3) to a year of

schooling until your son or daughter will be ultimately

toilet independence depending on the pace of learning

and teaching strategies applied by you.

CHAPTER 9

Ethics of Potty Training

Get Him or Her to Jump to Start with

Indicators

If your child is worked up about potty training and seems

to be getting the hang of it, or in case you have a dead

potty deadline you need to meet, you might help speed up

the procedure.

Select a day when you'll be home all day and will have

no outdoor engagement. Give your son or daughter lots

of salty snack foods and juice or drinking water or

beverage. Watch him or her cautiously for indicators to

pee or poo, or set a timer or maintain a log to ensure that

you keep in mind the approximate time to execute a potty

function every 30 mins. Make an effort to think of methods to make this a great event.

The ideology is that; taking more liquid in, means even more liquid out, so you should have lots of practice appointments to the toilet. And everybody knows that practice makes ideal perfection!

If your son or daughter spends time in someone else's care, make sure everyone communicates with one another relating to your child's potty teaching concept. Have a clear plan for potty training to ensure that everyone is constant whenever taking care of your child.

Be Prepared to Reach a Toilet Quickly

Even before your son or daughter asks, ensure that you always know where precisely the toilet is; if you are in a shop, a friend's house, or anywhere else. In this manner, you can move quickly whenever your child announces the necessity to go pee or poo.

A child who is not used to these potty lessons might wait before the last minute to announce his or her necessity to go pee or poo. Whenever your child says she's pressed, reach the potty and perform it quickly! While it's occasionally annoying to need to quit everything to consider taking him or her to the toilet, this is precisely everything you have wished to achieve. Your son or daughter recognizes the desire and delaying elimination until he or she reaches the toilet. So show patience and support, even though the urgent quest may cause you to quit whatever you are doing at the moment.

Potty Prize Giving Approach

Many parents have reported fantastic success with this vibrant idea. Here's how it operates:

- Purchase about thirty inexpensive little prizes. (Check the toy stores for an excellent collection of cheap trinkets.).

- Wrap each prize separately in colorful wrapping paper.

- Place the prizes in a clear plastic bowl on the toilet counter. You can call it the Potty Prize Treasure Package, or many other fun and enticing name.

- Tell your son or daughter, "They are potty prizes. You'll receive one every time you carry out your business in the toilet, simply with no hurry but whenever you're ready."

Most kids are "prepared" immediately, but you shouldn't be surprised if your son or daughter drools more than the prize bowl for some days before deciding to be ready.

Allow your kid to select one prize every time he or she will go. By enough time the prize bowl is certainly empty, the habit will end up being firmly set up. If your child requests a prize following the exhausting of the Treasure Packages, inquire to find a few of his or her aged awards and wrap them up once again. (Truly. The fun is generally in the unwrapping!)

After a while, your son or daughter will start to forget to require a prize, and you may quickly move to the "no-prize" phase.

Relax when Accidents Occur

Accidents are likely to happen during the training period. Utilize the same approach you utilize when she buttons her sweater the wrong manner or spills some milk. *"Oops. Missed the potty at that point. Don't worry, pretty soon you'll get it right."*

Accidents are incredibly normal, especially in the beginning of training. Nevertheless, if your son or daughter is having a lot more accidents than successes, or if either you or your son or daughter is getting distressed about these incidents, you might want to reconsider the readiness check to observe only if you've started a little too early.

Accidents are inevitable initially; however, they should steadily decrease. If indeed they continue after your son or daughter has completed training; nevertheless, you might need to examine the reason for them. If your son or daughter is just too busy to avoid her activity to access the toilet, perhaps you're in the best position to make it possible for him or her to recuperate from these episodes. You might like to get her more mixed up in the cleanup process. Train your child how precisely to help clean up any mess, change his or her personal clothing, and put her filthy pants in the laundry. If she's to help you look after all of this, it could help reduce these mishaps. It's typical for a kid to master taking care of potty schooling before another, so avoid being surprised of accidents happening for some time. Just maintain praising her successful attempts and keep focusing on the less-consistent process.

Offer Reward to Enhance Potty Learning

In case you are not sure that your son or daughter is physically ready for potty training, I'd advise against using any prize system. If he or she is physically unable to utilize the potty individually, you'll just be establishing him or her up for disappointment.

If, however, your child is set physically for potty schooling but is reluctant emotionally or adapting to the theory slowly, you might help spark the process with reward or "potty prizes." Regardless of what you've considered giving kids prizes as rewards previously, there are occasions to utilize this effective idea during potty teaching. According to some polls, a lot more than 80 percent of parents conform to giving their children benefits or prizes for using the potty so that you would be in good company.

Survey has revealed that most kids and preschoolers could be highly motivated to create adjustments when offered prizes-which, I'm sure, is an excellent surprise for you! There are many approaches you may use.

Duration of Encouragement

Some specialists say that you need to give a whole load of positive opinions, including a party-like atmosphere-actually with noisemakers, cake, and party hats. Others state that you ought to avoid getting overly thrilled or emotional and acknowledge that your son or daughter has done well. The proper answer is that the appropriate response is different for each parent and child pair. Some parents are naturally more thinking about everything their kids perform; others tend to be reserved.

Some women thrive on the parents' energy, and other kids are easily overwhelmed. Even two different kids in the same family will respond quickly to varying degrees of enthusiasm.

Probably the most excellent advice is to accomplish what comes naturally. What's most significant is that you would like your child to learn that you support him, that you will be pleased with his efforts and also his successes.

Patience

This whole process does take time. You almost certainly won't feel confident to completely start your son or daughter's toileting for most months. So relax, show patience, and revel in the journey. Kids are just little for a short time to embrace the training effectively.

CHAPTER 10

BED WETTING

When your son or daughter uses the toilet all day with only rare errors, you can think about your toilet training working effectively, even if your son or daughter still wears a diaper to bed. Nighttime dryness is an entirely separate subject.

Toilet schooling is accomplished whenever a child runs on the potty seat or toilet for bladder and bowel features during waking hours.

As children grow and develop, so carry out their ability to regulate their bladder. There is normally a wide variety of "normal" for whenever a kid achieves nighttime control. Bed-wetting, known as *enuresis*, is usually common amongst young children, with an increased percentage of males than girls. Because nearly half of most three-year-old's or more to 40 percent of four-year-old's wet the bed many times a week, it is considered normal behavior at these age groups. Additionally, 20 to 25 percent of five-year-old's and 10 to 15 percent of six-year-olds don't stay dry out every night.

By age nine, just 5 percent of children wet the bed, and the majority of those children do it only one time per month. As children grow older, few of them possess bed-wetting accidents. In nearly all cases, the issue goes away completely even when parents avoid any unique treatment for the problem, and with the tiny percentage of kids who do want help, treatment is not at all hard.

The most commonly known reasons for bed-wetting in a kid are because of his or her physiology. Your son or daughter's child kidney aren't sending a sign to his or her mind when asleep, the brain is as well profoundly sleeping to listen to the indicators, his or her bladder hasn't grown huge enough to include a full night's way to hold urine or his or her organ over-produces urine during the night. As kids grow, most of these conditions are self-corrected.

Bed-wetting can be hereditary, so if one or both parents had been a bed wetter, a kid has about an 80 percent chance of doing the same by bed wetting. Diabetes, food sensitivities (particularly to caffeine, milk products, fruit, and chocolate), some medications, or additional health conditions can influence nighttime bladder-control problems. On occasion, bed-wetting could be a sign of a rest disorder; therefore if your son or daughter exhibits other indications, such as snoring or restless sleep, you might want to investigate this possibility.

No kid chooses to awaken cold and wet. Bed-wetting almost never is really because a kid is lazy or disobedient. Exactly like understanding how to walk or understanding how to talk, there's an array of "normal," and, like other milestones, every child achieves nighttime dryness on his or her time schedule. There is no reason to hurry the process.

For a bed-wetting toddler or preschooler, the perfect solution is easy: *allow your son or daughter to rest for naps and evening time in a diaper, padded teaching trousers, or disposable absorbent underpants until he or*

she starts to remain dry during naps and forever long.

How to Know When to Stop Using Diaper

When your kid has been sleeping dry for a week or more, it might be safe to get one of these night time or nap without diapers. Be ready for occasional accidents. The good idea is to double-make the bed. (Make use of a waterproof pad atop the bed sheet, and cover this with a second sheet which can be quickly removed if your son or daughter wets at night.) Keep an extra pair of pajamas nearby.

Some children appear to learn whenever a diaper is on the bottoms and utilize it rather than building a night or early-morning hours visit to the toilet. If your son or daughter is day-time independent and you imagine that she could be prepared to go without a diaper when sleeping, go ahead and test it out if she's prepared. As an experiment, make your child proceed diaper-less, sleeping atop a waterproof pad and double-made bed, to observe how he or she responds. You (and she) may be amazed by a dry bottom level and a dried-out bed each morning.

How to Enhance Toddler Dryness

While you need to focus on nighttime dryness when your child reaches the toilet training age, you might help a child who would like to stay dry during the night by doing the following:

- Encourage sufficient daytime liquids, and limit liquids for a couple of hours before bedtime. You don't have to cut out juices completely, because this reduces the quantity of nighttime urine, it generally does not stop the reason for bed-wetting.

- Make several outings to the toilet before bed-time one at the start of your bedtime routine and again at the end, right before lights out. Make sure your son or daughter finishes emptying his or her bladder by calming on the toilet for 3 to 5 moments. An egg timer might help your child understand how long to sit. You will keep him, or her organized with chat, reading a book, or tell a tale. Make this an essential component of your bedtime program.

- Help to make sure that your son or daughter uses the potty frequently during the day, about every single two hours. This encourages regular bladder function and may help with nighttime dryness.

- Direct your son or daughter to utilize the bathroom, whether it's been two hours or if you see symptoms of the need, such as squirming, wiggling, crotch keeping, or dancing.

- Avoid providing any meals or drinks that become stimulants, such as for example, chocolate, sugars, and caffeine, particularly in the hours before bedtime.

- Avoid having your son or daughter wear diapers or absorbent pull-up to bed and make use of a particular mattress cover. Instead, absorbent jeans or diapers will often delay the standard development process just because a kid can't experience when urination happens, and it could also provide him a subconscious message that it is OK to urinate during bedtime because he's putting on his pull-up.

- Make use of positive reinforcement with a sticker chart to help your son or daughter monitor his or her success.

- Keep a night-light-ON, to make the way to the toilet well lit and present your son or daughter access to utilize the toilet at nighttime if he or she must. Simply the subconscious message can help.

- Avoid putting any blame on your child, and don't make him feel guilty or ashamed. Tell him that wetting while asleep is normal and can remember to change.

CHAPTER 11

Most Commonly Known Reasons for Potty Training Problems

- The child isn't ready (lacks the correct physical skills).

- The child isn't ready (emotionally, socially, or behaviorally).

- The child doesn't know very well what he or she's supposed to do (communication).

- The child is becoming too distracted with something else to value going potty.

- The kid is uninterested in training.

- The child can be fearful of, or unpleasant with some aspect of training.

- Existence of a power struggle between the child and the parent.

- There's too much tension and pressure surrounding the process.

- The mother or father has unrealistic expectations.

- The parent isn't carrying out a toilet training program; it's hit or miss.

- The parent isn't ready (lacks time, endurance, or desire to carry out the process).

- The mother or father and caregiver don't acknowledge the strategies involved and are sending mixed messages.

- The mother or father is confusing normal mishaps with failure.

- The routine doesn't match the child's elimination pattern.

- The strategy used doesn't match the child's learning style or personality.

- The strategy used doesn't fit the parent's personality or teaching design.

- There exists a physical or medical deterrent (such as constipation, disease, or uncontrolled allergies).

Another essential point to understand is that you could lead a kid to the potty; nevertheless, you can't help to make him or her fill it. That is your child's undertaking, not really yours. You can teach her, you can prepare the required tools, and you will maintain positivity and support, but maybe for the very first time in her life, the most excellent result is entirely in her power.

Potty training appears like a huge little bit of chocolate cake, with a part of ice cream. Sprinkled with chocolates! Maybe even more amazing.

Endeavor to examine the prior list of commonly known reasons for toilet teaching problems and make an effort to figure out which part of it are obtainable in the form of effective toileting mastery for your son or daughter. After you have a deal with one of those fundamental reasons, it'll open up your brain to all types of new solutions. Afterward, read over the topics that adhere to match your problems.

CHAPTER 12

Behavioural Influence on Potty Training

Firstly, I have to cover some ground on the subject of boundaries and limits; after that, I'll hit particular behaviors I've seen in potty schooling. Boundaries and limitations have a poor rap in parenting lately. They can appear mean or draconian or too authoritarian. Many parents don't have confidence in any consequence or discipline. I want to state outright: *I do not advocate, nor do I believe in hitting or beating a kid ever.*

This is most likely the trickiest issue addressed in this book separating out behavioral conduct from potty training. There exists a lot for your son or daughter to understand when potty teaching your children. Certainly, the first couple of days, and maybe actually the first couple of weeks, are filled with learning. Learning, naturally, requires making some errors and/or having some incidents. However, there exists a difference between learning and behavior or habit. When your kid is showing behavior, and after all of the poor variety, the behavior must be addressed.

You are potty training around two-year age range, and around the same time, you might see various other two-year-old behavior. This might well be the first time you are seeing your child act, but it's normal. The awful twos aren't only a cliché; they are real. Throughout normal development, your son or daughter must test limitations. It's his work. He needs to find out where the fence is, as they say. The reason your wall in your backyard is there is indeed not to make your child wander and get misplaced. Limits and boundaries will be the fence in your child's psyche. With them intact, just while in your backyard, your child feels safe and sound, knowing where he may go and may not go.

A trend in contemporary parenting is to assume that the kid is with the capacity of deciding good stuff for himself without having to be provided any boundaries or limits. That is not the case. I frequently look to the Montessori system for how exactly to allow children to make some decisions while also providing boundaries. Within a framework, the kids are absolved from making choices; however they are not free to carry out whatever it is they need.

The children all consume lunch collectively. You can't make a couple of kids get a snack in the fridge and leave this up to them to choose if they are hungry, it could lead to mayhem. The kids all go outside jointly, whether one is tired or not really. Our children need some fences. Within those fences, we can enable tremendous freedom.

What I see, both from my experience and in my work is that most of us parents have a problem with providing freedom within boundaries. In our quest to improve free-thinking, kids are not offered enough framework to allow them to feel safe.

I see kids raised with no limitations or boundaries who by enough time they are age five or six, are wild and incredibly hard to control. By this, after exhibiting out-of-control behavior, not that they must be "controllable" just like a puppet.

Imagine the stress your child would feel if you were driving, been at the backseat, and he or she has zero idea of where you were heading. I've extrapolated that idea even more. Imagine if your son or daughter were responsible for providing you the directions, and which you followed their instructions. Proceed left. Go right. No. Stop. Wow. You'd quickly be lost, yes? That's where points will get mucky with the oft-touted child-led style of parenting. You could be child-led for the reason that you pay attention to and validate your son or daughter's opinion, but you just can't follow your child's lead through life. Both of you will get dropped. *The automobile you are driving is usually life, and it's your task to learn where you are going.* Ironically, most of the parents I've known in my own personal life are striving to give the youngster a "freedom" childhood. Still, how free is your son or daughter if he's entirely responsible for the direction the automobile is traveling. It's hugely anxiety-provoking. A free childhood ought to be about chocolate or vanilla, and something else.

All this is especially true in case you have a spirited or strong-willed child. I frequently work with parents who have a kid fitting this explanation. This child is generally demanding and will be challenging with regards to potty training as well. Still, this child requires boundaries and limits just as much as, or even more than, your garden-variety child.

All well and great, but what does this need to do with potty training?

Well, occasionally behavior kicks up during potty teaching. And because potty schooling is so wrought with emotion, it becomes hard to draw it aside from behavior. I also discover that parents will endure all types of behavior during potty schooling that they wouldn't work in other circumstances.

For example, one of the primary challenges parents today encounter during potty training gets their child to take a seat on the potty. Yes, you can go through to them or sing to them. I state it's alright to play with a mobile device seeing that as a distraction in the beginning. But, when you inquire your son or daughter to sit to go potty, your son or daughter should sit. Today, to a lot of individuals that sounds severe.

You show your son or daughter to sit and they don't. *How can you handle that?*

I'm requesting because-whatever your response is, that's how you're likely to handle it during potty training. When it's supper, it's time to sit and consume. When it's potty period, it's time to take a seat on the potty.

Once you encounter behavior during potty training, do your very best to put it right into a different context. That will assist you to figure out how better to deal with it in the context of potty schooling. It's your parenting duty. I do not really nor have I ever comfy telling people the way to handle behavior generally. That's why I'm providing you a framework to work with, and you may make your own parenting decisions.

Many parents say, "We don't feel safe making him sit." I agree. I don't believe you should force your son or daughter to sit. Nevertheless, it's worth pondering precisely how fearful we are because of the potty. Many parents dread doing anything unfavorable around potty training. Utilizing a firm or stern voice seems contrary to these parents, and they're worried about traumatizing the kid. This is where another scenario will come in handy. Everyone has held their kid down and strapped them in the car seat. Even though they are kicking, screaming, and hitting. We perform it because we should go somewhere, and we need them to be safe. Has your son or daughter ever been traumatized by that rather than wished to sit in the automobile front seat someday? I'm guessing No. Again, I'm not saying you should exert pressure on your child onto the potty or strap him down, or anything remotely like this. I'm simply pointing out that fear of traumatizing a kid by conveying the message that you mean business has gotten a bit out of control.

Another thing to bear in mind may be the difference between *"the kid you have" and "the kid you want."* You have a child you have, definitely not the kid you need. This is also true during potty training.

I can give you recommendations about any special conditions you might have, but we can not change your zebra's stripes. Still, that is hard for all of us to admit and hard to keep in mind. Most of us want the well-behaved,

loving, courteous kid. We got what we want. Still, our choice is fierce. When you are potty training, take care not to linger in the property of "I want him . . ." We can deal with what we have, but we can not cope with fantasy.

There's another aspect to "a child you have." If your son or daughter shows a particular "problem"- say he's whiny, or she's resistant or susceptible to histrionics and tantrums, you will have this same kid if you are potty teaching. No judgment; there is absolutely no behavior I've not really seen. Still, I discover parents who in some way think potty training will happen in a bubble-that the rest of the behavior the kid exhibits is somehow not likely to appear even though it's potty training. That is a big transition, so these behaviors can not only be right there, but they may get magnified for a brief period. Again, it's all great. Just keep your anticipations level as well as your love big.

Whatever your child's personality is, I can't change that or correct it; that's built-in the child's physiology. If your son or daughter is exhibiting the behavior you do not like, or you are feeling is usually disrespectful, you will likely see that same behavior during potty schooling. What I could tell you is how exactly to deal with a few of the behaviors you find in potty training.

Here's a clear exemplary case of behavior. Say your son or daughter did ideal for a couple of days. Suddenly, she doesn't want to utilize the potty anymore. This may appear to be a defiant "NO!" or it could seem she just can't be bothered with this. If she sat and peed/pooped on the potty several time, then we realize she can perform it, it's that easy. If she subsequently chooses never to, it's behavior.

In case you are feeling unfortunate or just a little heartbroken that it isn't heading as you intended, it's likely that your son or daughter needs more learning. If you feel as if you are being pranked, if you feel anger, or if you feel like strangling your kid, I'll wager it's behavior. Usually, parents have a pervasive sense when they are coping with behavior but don't carry out anything because they're terrified of "traumatizing" the kid.

Having boundaries and pursuing through won't traumatize your kid in any sense. When you have a youngster who you understand is taking part in you, the very best move to make is provide a small, instant, appropriate consequence. For example, take away the play toy he was using when he wet his slacks, or consider restraining him from the activity where he was involved.

Toddlers don't have that extended way of thinking. For this reason, sticker charts are ineffective. Toddlers don't have the thought process to state, "Wow. I've six stickers; yet another and I'll have a week of staying dry out!"

The small, immediate consequence can be helpful when you aren't sure whether he needs more learning or is exhibiting the behavior. I believe I've managed to get clear that satisfaction and self-mastery ought to be the motivation behind potty training a child effectively. However, for a few children that by no means clicks in, plus they need some exterior motivation to nudge things along. Some parents react such as, "But I'll feel terrible if I provide him a consequence, and he needs even more learning." Removing a little toy consequently won't scar your child forever. And it's the quickest way to get a remedy. If your child can't utilize the potty realizing that his toy is sure to get placed on the fridge for one hour if he doesn't, you can wager that so far he needs more to learn, and he won't be scared. If your child can do it all, you then know the incidents are because of behavior. I'm talking about real-world potty training, not theory. Effects are sure to get you your solution the fastest.

Some parents say, "Isn't a consequence only the opposite of an incentive? I'd rather give incentive for the behavior I want rather than provide a consequence for what We don't want." I am aware of the idea behind this and, yes, generally, positive reinforcement is most effective with children. Nevertheless, we get back to that notion of expected behavior. The problem with benefits and potty schooling is that they get sticky. The stakes must be continuously raised to ensure they work. If you are likely to reward for peeing, where else can that lead? I'd rather curb undesired behavior than prize the hell out of excellent behavior. Else, you finish up with a youngster who expects to end up being rewarded for everything.

I fully have confidence in benefits for exemplary behavior, and I also think that bad behavior gets a consequence.

Dedication

This book is dedicated to all loving parents in the world.

Quote!

The problem is not the problem, but

the problem is actually how you handle

the problem

Printed in the USA
CPSIA information can be obtained
at www.ICGtesting.com
LVHW041547200224
772364LV00008B/162